# SCABIES

## Skin Health for Life: Understanding Scabies for Dermatological Resilience

**CHAD BRUNO**

# Table of Contents

## Introductory

The mite Sarcoptes scabiei is responsible for the highly contagious skin condition known as scabies. In order to lay its eggs and produce acute itching, this tiny mite digs into the skin's outermost layer. Scabies is primarily transmitted through close physical contact, such as touching the skin of an infected person, and it is more likely in crowded or close living settings, such families, schools, and nursing facilities.

• Itching, especially at night, a rash with small, pimple-like lumps, and the development of tiny, thread-like burrows on the skin are common symptoms of scabies. Wrists, finger joints, elbows, armpits, stomach, and genitalia are the most typical sites of infection.

• Prescription drugs, mainly topical creams or lotions that kill the mites and their eggs, can be used to treat scabies. In order to prevent reinfection, all close contacts of the infected individual should be treated, regardless of whether or not they exhibit symptoms. Seek medical help if you think you have scabies or have had close contact with someone who does, so the

condition may be properly
diagnosed and treated.

# CHAPTER ONE
## Structure and Development

Understanding the scabies infestation and its transmission requires an understanding of the anatomy and lifecycle of the scabies mite, Sarcoptes scabbier. The following is a summary of its structure and development:

## Sarcoptes Scabies Anatomy:

**1.** Sarcoptes scabies mites are so tiny that they are nearly invisible to the naked eye, reaching about 0.3 to 0.4 millimeters in length.

**2.** The mite has a spherical body, four legs, and a tiny, pointed head.

It can penetrate the skin because of its shape.

**3.** The cuticle is a tough outer coat that protects the mite's soft body.

• Mite eggs are normally laid in a tunnel the female mite has dug into the skin's outermost layer. The eggs are roughly 0.15 millimeters in size and have an oval shape.

• **Larva:** The eggs develop into larvae after a few days. These juvenile mites are more agile due to their six legs.

• **Eight-legged nymph:** The larvae's next stage of development. Over the course of a week or so, the nymphs develop into full-grown mites.

• **Adult:** Adult mites are the most active and can move quickly from one host to another, mate, and produce new generations of mites.

It takes roughly two to four weeks for the creature to mature from an egg to an adult. As the mites burrow into the skin and lay eggs, the infected person experiences severe itching and a rash. Most of the burrowing and egg-laying is done by the female mites, whereas the males are much smaller and less active.

The extreme itching and redness are caused by an allergic reaction to the mites, their eggs, and their waste products, and can be spread through close human contact. Prescription drugs, usually in the form of topical creams or lotions, are used to treat scabies by destroying the mites and their eggs.

## Dissemination and Propagation

Close contact with an infected person is the most common way to catch scabies. Scabies is contagious because the mite Sarcoptes scabiei can jump from person to person. Common routes of scabies transmission include:

• The most common way scabies is spread from one person to another is through direct skin-to-skin contact. Whenever two people are in close proximity to one another, whether by embracing, holding hands, sexual contact, or otherwise, this is what happens.

• Scabies is highly contagious and can quickly spread between members of the same household or between intimate partners. Transmission can occur through the exchange of infected personal objects such as bedding, clothing, towels, etc.

• Due to close quarters and the sharing of personal things, scabies can easily spread among youngsters in childcare and school settings. Infestations are commonplace in such conditions.

• Healthcare institutions: Scabies can also be transmitted within healthcare institutions, including hospitals and nursing homes, especially in settings where there is close patient contact.

• Scabies epidemics are more likely to happen in confined, institutional settings like prisons and homeless shelters, where people often share sleeping quarters and have limited access to showers and other hygienic amenities.

• Since scabies mites can infest the vaginal and pubic areas, they can be spread through sexual contact. It is a type of STI (sexually transmitted illness).

• While it is not very common, fomite transmission can occur when a mite lives on an inanimate object such as a piece of furniture or a piece of clothes for an extended period of time. These goods can be spread if they come into contact with an infected person's personal effects.

Avoiding intimate contact with infected people, not sharing personal things, and engaging in safe sex are all effective ways to limit the spread of scabies. A person with scabies should get medical treatment to get rid of the mites and stop spreading the disease. To stop the spread of the infestation within the family or neighborhood, close friends and family members may also need to be medicated.

# CHAPTER TWO
## Infection-Predisposing Factors

The likelihood of contracting scabies is influenced by a number of variables. Individuals with these risk factors may be more likely to become infected. Scabies risk factors include, among others:

• The most important risk factor for contracting scabies is having close, persistent skin-to-skin contact with an infected person. This includes making physical touch with another person, such as in a hug or holding hands.

## 2. Household or Family Contact:
Living in close quarters with an

infested person, such as within the same household or family, increases the risk, as it allows for simple transmission of mites through shared items and proximity.

• Because of the tight quarters and shared amenities, scabies thrives in institutional and crowded living environments including dorms, prisons, shelters, and nursing homes.

• Attendance at a daycare or school raises a child's risk because of the frequent close contact and sharing of personal goods that occurs there.

- Nurses and other healthcare workers may be at increased risk of contracting scabies from patients because of their close proximity to them during an outbreak.

- Contact between an infected person and a sexual partner can spread scabies, especially if the genital or pubic areas are afflicted.

- People with compromised immune systems may be more prone to scabies and may experience more severe infestations. These people include those with HIV/AIDS, cancer, or certain autoimmune illnesses.

• In tight quarters such as those found in nursing homes and other types of long-term care, scabies can thrive among the elderly.

• An increased risk of reinfection exists for people who have had scabies in the past and come into touch with an infected person.

• The danger of contracting a mite infestation is greatly increased if you share clothing, bedding, towels, or other personal items with someone who already has one.

Scabies can infect persons of any age or socioeconomic status. Avoiding direct contact with infected people and not sharing personal goods are two ways to lessen your chances of becoming scabies. If you have any of these risk factors and start experiencing scabies symptoms, it is crucial that you contact a doctor right away.

## Symptoms and Indicators

Symptoms of a scabies infestation vary, but the most typical ones are:

• Scabies are characterized by acute itching, which is particularly bothersome at night. Because of an allergic reaction to mites, their eggs, and their waste products, you're experiencing intense itching.

• Rash Small, red, raised lumps or pimple-like lesions are the hallmark of a scabies rash. The rash may develop widely and manifest in a wide variety of places on the body.

• Scabies mites dig extremely fine, threadlike burrows just below the skin's surface. These burrows may appear as little, elevated, grayish-white, or skin-colored lines or tracks. Common locations include the creases of the skin, such as the crooks of the fingers, the underside of the arms, and the vaginal area.

• The skin may develop pustules (fluid-filled blisters) or vesicles (small fluid-filled sacs) if scabies is present.

• Scratching the extremely itching regions can cause the skin to split, which in turn might invite subsequent bacterial infections. Increased redness, heat, swelling, and the appearance of pus are all possible outcomes.

• **Crusty lesions:** People with compromised immune systems are more likely to develop sores or crusty lesions after a scabies infestation. This is the more severe and contagious form of scabies known as crusted (Norwegian) scabies.

- Less frequently, and more typically in the case of crusted scabies, a person with scabies may feel more generalized symptoms, such as fever and exhaustion.

It's crucial to understand that the signs and symptoms of scabies might differ from person to person. Some people may experience no symptoms at all from an infestation, while others may suffer from intense itching and other skin abnormalities.

If you or someone you know exhibits any of these symptoms, it is crucial to contact a doctor for a diagnosis and treatment of scabies.

Early detection and treatment of scabies can stop the progress of the infestation and its effects. In order to stop the spread of the disease, close contacts may also need to be tested and treated.

# CHAPTER THREE
## Examining and Diagnosing

Clinical examination and sometimes laboratory testing are used together to determine a scabies diagnosis.

**1. Clinical Assessment:** First, the doctor will do a complete physical examination. Scabies can be identified by its telltale rash, burrows, and extreme itching, so they'll be on the lookout for them. In addition to asking about symptoms, the doctor will inquire about the patient's health background, recent interactions, and potential scabies exposure.

**2.** The healthcare provider may use a dermatoscope or magnifying lens to inspect the patient's skin and look for signs of burrows or mites. These tunnels tend to appear in creases of skin, like those around the fingers, wrists, elbows, armpits, and genitalia.

**3.** A skin scraping or biopsy may be performed if the diagnosis is in doubt or if the presence of scabies mites needs to be confirmed. This method involves extracting a small piece of skin from the afflicted region and examining it under a microscope to look for evidence of mites, eggs, or excrement. This is known as a skin scrape or skin biopsy.

**4.** An ink test may be used to help make a diagnosis by a doctor in specific situations. To do this, dab some ink onto the spot and wipe it clean. It's possible that the ink becomes trapped in the mites' burrows, highlighting them.

**5.** In order to diagnose scabies, doctors often employ a procedure called dermoscopy, which involves the use of a specialized equipment to inspect the skin in greater detail.

**6.** Family and close friends may be asked about their exposure to the patient in order to gauge the severity of the infection and whether or not they need to be tested or treated themselves.

A clinical diagnosis of scabies is usually accurate and confirmatory laboratory testing is not necessarily required. However, in some circumstances where the diagnosis is questionable or when scabies is suspected in persons with atypical presentations, skin scrapings or biopsies can offer definite confirmation.

Prescription drugs, mainly topical creams or lotions that kill the mites and their eggs, are typically recommended for treatment of scabies by medical professionals. It is vital to follow the specified treatment regimen and take efforts to prevent reinfestation, including washing and drying contaminated bedding and clothing and informing close contacts for evaluation and potential treatment.

## Cases of Scabies

Scabies infestations can manifest in a number of various ways, and the condition itself has a number of variants and subtypes.

- Intense itching, a rash of little red bumps, and the presence of burrows on the skin are all hallmarks of classic scabies, the most prevalent form of the skin condition. Anyone of any age can get the classic form of scabies.

• Crusted scabies, often known as Norwegian scabies, is a very contagious and painful type of the skin ailment. Crusty scabies is characterized by scaly lesions covered in a thick crust and a high mite count. People with compromised immune systems, such as those with HIV/AIDS, cancer, or certain autoimmune illnesses, are more likely to contract this subtype.

- Firm, irritating nodules or lumps develop under the skin in a disease called nodular scabies, a less frequent type of the disorder. These nodules may be present long after the scabies infection has been successfully treated.

- Rarely, a scabies infestation can cause fluid-filled blisters or vesicles to grow on the skin, a condition known as bullous scabies.

- Infantile scabies is a form of scabies that primarily affects babies and toddlers. A rash from scabies can appear anywhere on a baby's body, including the palms, soles, and face.

• Most cases of senile scabies occur in the elderly. It may present as scaly, itchy lesions, and it might be more chronic in this age group.

• When a person with scabies utilizes topical steroids (such as corticosteroid treatments) to alleviate itching, they are said to have scabies incognito. Scabies is difficult to diagnose since corticosteroids temporarily hide the disease's outward signs. However, this method of treatment may hasten the mites' spread.

Although the Sarcoptes scabiei mite is responsible for all of these variations, the severity and clinical presentation of the disease can vary greatly from one form to the next. Prescription medication is often used to eradicate the mites in these variants, albeit the specific method may differ according to the subtype and the individual's health status. Scabies can be managed and its problems avoided with prompt identification and treatment.

# CHAPTER FOUR
## Choices in Medical Care

Prescription drugs that are effective against Sarcoptes scabiei mites and their eggs are commonly used to treat scabies. The standard methods for dealing with scabies are as follows:

## 1. Creams and lotions that kill scabies on contact:

• The most popular and efficient scabicide is permethrin cream. A full application is made from the neck down and then kept on for 8-14 hours before being washed off. Most people put it on before going to bed. The typical treatment cycle for this modality is 7 days.

The topical scabicide ivermectin cream may also be utilized in some situations.

**2.** It's possible that your doctor will recommend oral ivermectin if you've tried other therapies without success. It is usually administered as a single dose followed by another dose a week later.

### 3. Close Relatives Care:

- All close contacts (family members, sexual partners, roommates) should be treated for scabies, regardless of whether or not they show symptoms. For best results, they should both take part in the same treatment program.

**4.** Itching can be treated with antihistamines, which are sometimes recommended but do not kill the mites. Diphenhydramine and other nonprescription antihistamines can also help reduce scratching.

**5.** Symptomatic relief can be achieved with the use of cold baths, cold compresses, or over-the-counter anti-itch creams or lotions (such as hydrocortisone), as prescribed by a doctor.

**6.** All clothing, bedding, and towels used in the two days before to starting treatment should be washed in hot water and dried on high heat to prevent reinfestation. Mites can be killed by vacuum sealing an item for at least 72 hours in a plastic bag. Mattresses and upholstered furniture should especially be vacuumed.

**7.** Measures to Prevent Reinfestation in the Environment Vacuuming and cleaning the home may be required. But scabies mites can't make it very far away from a human host.

It is crucial to stick to the treatment plan exactly as it was laid out by a doctor. In order to completely eradicate the problem, it is often advised to repeat the therapy after some time has passed. For the same reason, it's important to limit interaction with people while taking treatment. If symptoms persist or worsen following therapy, a follow-up with a healthcare provider is recommended.

Any severe or unexpected symptoms, or any worries about the treatment, should be reported to the doctor. To stop the spread of scabies, close contacts should be notified and kept under observation for symptoms and signs of infestation.

## Avoiding Scratches

Avoiding direct contact with Sarcoptes scabiei mites is crucial for preventing a scabies infestation. The following are some precautions to take:

### 1. Maintain Proper Hygiene

• Wash your hands often with soap and water, but especially after coming into close contact with people who may have scabies.

Do your best to prevent the spread of disease by practicing good hygiene and keeping a clean environment.

## 2. Stay Away From Each Other

• Avoid prolonged, close skin-to-skin contact with people who have scabies or who you fear may have scabies.

Hugging, holding hands, and other forms of physical contact with an infected person should be avoided.

**3. Never lend out your personal belongings:**

• Don't let people who have scabies borrow your clothes, towels, sheets, or personal care products like razors or combs.

**4. Cleaning and drying infested items:**

• Wash and dry any clothing, bedding, and towels used within the previous two days before beginning treatment in hot water and high heat if you have had contact with someone who has scabies. If there were any mites on these goods, they would die.

The best way to get rid of mites on items that can't be washed is to put them in a plastic bag for at least three days.

## 5. Use Safe Sexual Behavior:

• If you are sexually active and one partner has scabies, it's crucial to use protection (condoms) to prevent the transfer of the mites.

## 6. Keep your distance in potentially dangerous situations:

• Take extra precautions with personal hygiene and avoid direct contact with people in crowded or institutional settings including dorms, hospitals, nursing homes, and homeless shelters.

## 7. Maintenance Exams:

• People in high-risk occupations or environments, such as those in healthcare or in institutions, should get regular exams and be on the lookout for scabies symptoms.

## 8. Get Emergency Care:

• Seek medical help for diagnosis and treatment if you think you have scabies or have had close contact with someone who does. If the infestation is treated quickly, it can be contained.

Scabies is a medical problem that can be effectively treated and controlled with the right care. The spread of scabies can be stopped if it is diagnosed and treated quickly. Furthermore, it is crucial to treat all close contacts simultaneously when scabies is discovered in a family or tight-knit community to prevent reinfestation.

## Managing Scabbing Itch

Although scabies and the accompanying itching and discomfort can be difficult to deal with, there are things you can do to alleviate your suffering.

• Visit a Doctor for Diagnosis and TreatmentSeeing a doctor for a diagnosis and treatment is the first and most crucial step. Scabicides, drugs used to kill mites, will be prescribed to alleviate the infestation.

• To get the best results from your therapy, it's important to strictly adhere to your doctor's orders. A second treatment, possibly after a week, may be necessary to guarantee that all mites are eradicated. This may involve applying a topical scabicide or taking oral medication.

- The itching that can occur during treatment needs to be managed. Your doctor may advise you to use over-the-counter antihistamines or topical treatments (such as hydrocortisone) to alleviate the itch. Scratching can cause more skin injury and infection.

- The risk of skin damage from scratching can be reduced by maintaining appropriate personal hygiene habits including taking frequent showers and cutting fingernails short.

- Items that were worn or used within the last two days should be washed and dried in hot water and high heat to eliminate any remaining mites. Put the items in a plastic bag and leave them sealed for at least 72 hours if they can't be washed.

• Staying away from close quarters with other people is essential during treatment, especially in high-risk settings. Share this news with your loved ones so they can get checked out and treated if needed.

• Vacuum your home thoroughly, paying special attention to the mattress and upholstered furniture. Although scabies mites cannot survive for long away from the host, reinfestation can be prevented with proper hygiene.

• If you want to stop the spread of scabies, it's important to take care of your close contacts and family members.

• After treatment, it's important to keep an eye out for any lingering symptoms or new signs of infestation. If you experience a reinfestation, get quick medical assistance.

• Educate yourself on scabies and how to avoid getting it to lessen the likelihood of future outbreaks.

Dealing with scabies can be challenging, but it can be efficiently controlled with the right therapy and consistent follow-up care. Even if your symptoms improve before the end of therapy, it is still important to finish the full course of medication as suggested by your doctor. Do not be shy about consulting your doctor if you have any concerns or questions about your condition or its treatment.

## Conclusion

The Sarcoptes scabiei mite is the infectious agent in scabies. It causes severe itching, manifests as a rash of tiny red bumps, and is accompanied by the appearance of tiny burrows on the skin. Scabies is a contagious skin disease that can be spread from person to person. Different clinical manifestations are seen in the many scabies subtypes, such as classic scabies, crusted scabies, nodular scabies, and bullous scabies.

- In most situations, laboratory testing is used to corroborate a clinical diagnosis of scabies.

Scabicide drugs, such as oral and topical creams and lotions, are available by prescription to treat scabies. It is crucial to follow the suggested treatment regimen properly and take preventive steps to avoid reinfestation.

• Safe sex practices, regular showers, not touching infected people, and not sharing personal belongings are all ways to reduce your risk of contracting scabies. Seeking timely medical treatment, dealing with itching, maintaining excellent cleanliness, and preventing the spread of the infection to close contacts are all important parts of coping with scabies.

Scabies is manageable and can be controlled with the right treatment and by following doctor's orders. It is important to see a doctor if you think you have scabies or have any questions or concerns about the illness.

**THE END**

www.ingramcontent.com/pod-product-compliance
Lightning Source LLC
Chambersburg PA
CBHW060811260726
48660CB00002B/890